NON-ALCOHOLIC DRINKS

EASY-TO-DO INTERNATION BEVERAGES!

By Drew Liddle

About the author

Dr. Drew Liddle B.A., Ph.D., is the author of numerous textbooks and of seven works of popular fiction; he has also taught school, been a university lecturer, a journalist, theatre critic, jazz musician, adman and, most recently, a management consultant.

Many of the recipes in this book were collected by Drew Liddle on his professional travels on four continents. He has broadcast widely on the subject of drinks and written numerous articles. For this book, he has opened up the notebooks he compiled over more than a quarter of a century.

About this book

This easy-to-read, unfussy, hugely informative book is written on the basis there are no rules for concocting sensational drinks and very often the stated ingredients in any recipe can be played around with. Doing so might well produce a better drink. Have fun, be creative and make your own as well as the ones in this book. You don't have to be an expert and very many of the drinks can be made in five minutes or less, following the easy step-by-step instructions. Generally you need no other equipment than a blender.

And there's a whole range of different types of drinks, one for every week of the year - to help you choose something right for that special occasion, cure a hangover, act as a tonic, as well as just tickle your taste buds and refresh you.

If you are hosting a party or throwing a summer barbeque, taking a drink by the pool or just enjoying a quiet summer day, these recipes are sure to delight all members of the family.

But if it's cold outside this book is also for you. In fact, whatever the weather, whatever the occasion and whatever your mood, you will find the selections here particularly useful. They are arranged in no particular order so this is a book which is great for browsing – and there's one drink for every week of the year!

You will find the 'talking points' - in which the author shares information and ideas picked up over a lifetime in the trade - particularly informative and insightful. As are the introductions to famous branded drinks, like Badoit, Malta, Kracherl, L&P, that you may not be familiar with but are likely to find deliciously refreshing, and which can be bought on line. Then there's those handy hints on how to garnish the drinks and present them looking at their best.

Maybe best of all are the insights into some of the world's most famous bars, restaurants and hotels, where many of these drinks, particularly the cocktails, were first consumed - in places as far flung as Barcelona, Milan, New York, Delhi and Melbourne.

Of course, how the bar staff made these delicious drinks is their secret but this book is the next best thing to being there and sampling one yourself, and each recipe has been tried and tested, to provide a source of endless delight for your palate.

So next time you find yourself simply reaching for the Koolaid powder, don't! Here is what you've been waiting for if you're teetotal or just want some heavenly-tasting, health-giving drinks that aren't going to damage your liver. In fact, far from damaging any part of you, most of them will be of great value to your mind and body. Most of them are ideal for children, too.

And if you absolutely can't do without your alcohol very many of them can be spiced up by a dash of vodka, gin or rum to produce wonderfully inventive cocktails.

1 - PLUM AND GINGER JIVE

I first drank this in the delightful surroundings of The Brewery, Mildura, Victoria, Australia, where I'd actually gone to review the rather fine range of beers they produce. The area is famous for the deliciousness of its plums and I was served this drink to clean my palate, with fruit that had been picked that morning. A never-to-be forgotten experience!

Serving:

- Makes 2 glasses

Ingredients:

- 2 ripe plums, skin on, chopped
- 3 cups water
- 1 tablespoon fresh ginger, peeled and sliced
- 3/4 cup sugar
- 330 mls club soda

Instructions:

- Bring water to boil
- Toss in chopped plums, reduce heat, and simmer until plums are cooked and mushy and the liquid is bright red, about 15 to 20 minutes
- In the last 5 minutes of simmering, toss in ginger slices
- Turn off heat and stir in sugar until fully dissolved
- Let cool. Strain liquid and discard solids
- Add ice cubes to each glass and fill with plum syrup to two thirds of the way
- Top with club soda, give each glass a stir, and serve

Talking Points:

- The most time-consuming part is quarter of an hour spent cooking down the plums and throwing in the ginger slices, and the 20 minutes or so the liquid takes to cool. Then just strain, top with soda, and serve over ice
- Why is it called Plum and Ginger Jive? Well just try it and you'll want to start bopping!

2 - LEMON SQUASH

I was served something like this basic recipe in The Marshmallow, in Moreton-in-Marsh - a delightful English tea-room in one of the most unspoiled areas of England, the Cotswolds. It seemed so archetypally English that I almost asked for cucumber sandwiches!

Serving:

- Makes a bottle

Ingredients:

- 3 lemons minced or blended
- 30 g of citric acid
- 2 kilos sugar
- 2.5 ltrs boiling water

Instructions:

- Bring lemons to boil in the water
- Turn off heat and add sugar and citric acid
- Stir until both are dissolved
- Allow to cool and then bottle
- Dilute with cold water to taste and decorate with a sprig of mint

Talking Point:

- A tangy, refreshing drink made from a classic recipe and ideal for all the family on a hot summer's day

3 - BERRY BLISS

I drank the best version of this ever at a bar in Heidelberg, the Sonderbar, a wonderful watering hole in this charming university town, where I found students and professors cheek by jowl, tourists and workaday folk all happily socialising.

Serving:

- Makes 4 glasses

Ingredients:

- 300 g fresh strawberries (use 4 for decorating)
- 150 g fresh blueberries
- 2 bananas
- 300 mls vanilla yoghurt (strawberry yoghurt can be used if preferred)
- 10 g clear honey (this can be omitted or increased according to taste)

Instructions:

- Wash the strawberries, raspberries and blueberries
- Put into a blender along with the other ingredients, adding the honey when the fruit is smooth before another little blending
- Pour into 4 glasses and decorate with a strawberry

Talking Point:

- Ummm! Nice! How refreshing, wholesome and healthy

4 - CARROT AND ORANGE COCKTAIL

Serving:

- Makes one cocktail

Ingredients:

- 2 medium-sized oranges, peeled and segmented
- 450 g carrots
- Seasoning to taste

Instructions:

- Peel carrots and process them with oranges in juice extractor
- Mix together well, and season to taste

Talking Point:

- This is a simple and extremely health-giving little drink, ideal for breakfast

5 - SPARKLING FRUITS OF THE FOREST

I came upon this refreshing drink at an old Black Forest gasthof, in Freiburg, Germany, which prided itself on making the best Black Forest cake – but was certainly entitled to make the same claim for this drink, as I recall. I sat on the terrace looking out over the town with sun going down and the lights coming on - wondering why life couldn't always be this good.

Serving:

- Makes enough for a party

Ingredients:

- 350 g mixed berries - strawberries, red currants, raspberries blackberries, blackcurrants
- 1 orange – garnish

- 600 mls lemonade

Instructions:

- Process fruits in juice extractor
- Mix juices with the lemonade
- Garnish with kiwi fruit and serve over ice cubes

Talking Point:

- These berries are an amazing source of antioxidants, to keep you strong and healthy by fighting the free radicals that are trying to harm you

6 - SIMA MEAD

I've never been to Finland, alas, but got this recipe from a colleague who had and came back full of the joys of spring having sampled this delicious beverage.

Serving:

- 4 ltrs

Ingredients:

- 4 ltrs water
- 250 g soft brown sugar (firmly packed)
- 250 g regular white sugar
- 1½ - 2 lemons
- 1/8 tsp fresh yeast
- Raisins

Instructions:

- Pour the sugars in a clean, large glass jar rinsed with boiling water. If the brown sugar you are using is very dark or strong in flavour, and if you want the mead to be lighter in colour and taste, replace some of the brown sugar with white sugar
- Wash and brush the lemons under hot running water. In thin strips, peel out their yellow zest, place in a strainer and rinse with boiling water. Halve the peeled lemons and squeeze out their juice. Bring the water to the boil and pour about half of it on the sugars in the jar. After the sugar has melted, add the lemon juice and zest
- Let the mixture stand until it is lukewarm. Also let the other half of water cool until lukewarm. Dissolve the yeast in a small amount of the water and add to the lukewarm sugar mixture along with the rest of the lukewarm water. Stir thoroughly, cover with a loose lid or cloth and let stand overnight at room temperature
- The mixture should begin to ferment within a day. Strain the mixture through a fine cheesecloth and pour in sterilized bottles. Add about 1 teaspoon sugar and 5 - 10 raisins in every bottle. Raisins can be omitted. Close the bottles with tight-fitting caps
- Let the mead bottles stand at room temperature for about 3 hours before transferring to a cold cellar or

refrigerator. The fermentation will continue in the bottles so store them cold, or else the pressure building inside the bottles may break them. For this reason, do not exceed the amount of yeast given in the recipe
- The mead will be drinkable, after about ten days, as soon as the raisins in the bottles have risen to the surface, but the taste improves with storage
- Serve with sugared funnel cake, if you want to finnish (!) the job properly

Talking Points:

- This sparkling mead is the May Day drink in Finland and very good it is on any day of the year
- Mead made according to this ancient and traditional way is virtually non-alcoholic and is suitable for children
- Make sure you sterilize with boiling water all the equipment you will use: jars, lids, cheesecloth, saucepans, spoons, funnels, bottles, caps etc.
- This is, obviously, one of the most time-consuming recipes in the book – but the product is certainly worth the effort! It tastes like the distillation of spring itself!

7 - CHOCOLATE COFFEE DELIGHT

I experienced a variant of this - and it is an experience in itself - in the Hard Rock Café, in the centre of New York's Times Square, surrounded by a fantastically evocative collection of Rock iconography, which brought my youth back to me. It was an amazing afternoon of nostalgia served up with the sort of richly velvety drink that was the perfect complement.

Serving:

- Makes two mugs

Ingredients:

- 300 mls semi-skimmed milk
- 4 teaspoons good quality instant coffee
- 2 teaspoons drinking chocolate
- 2 tablespoons double cream

- Add whipped cream to taste and decorate with chocolate curls

Instructions:

- Heat milk
- Whisk in the coffee and drinking chocolate
- Bring to nearly boiling point and then pour into cups
- Pour the cream over the back of a metal spoon and the cream will float on top
- Sprinkle with chocolate curls

Talking Point:

- Definitely not part of a slimmer's diet – but delightful for a bout of self-indulgence, which now and then can do you a lot of good

8 - SINFUL COFFEE

I drank the best ever, actually, when I stopped by Marylou's, in Lucerne, California, on my way to Lake County. Which only goes to show you don't have to be dining at the Ritz to get the best!

Serving:

- Makes two cups

Ingredients:

- 300 mls water
- 1 tablespoon good quality coffee
- 1 tablespoon sugar
- 2 cinnamon sticks
- Double cream, whisked.

Instructions:

- Heat water, coffee, sugar and cinnamon sticks in pan until it boils
- Remove from heat for quarter of a minute, and bring to boil twice more
- Strain into cups
- Serve black or with the whisked cream spooned onto the top

Talking Points:

- Another bout of self-indulgence today. Why not!
- You may have heard of the Cinnamon Challenge, an internet-inspired cult that requires the silly participant to swallow – or try to – a tablespoonful of cinnamon in less than a minute. Don't bother because the cinnamon quickly dries on the tongue stopping you swallowing
- Instead take your sweet and spicy cinnamon in this drink. It blends beautifully with the coffee and cream. And what a heady aroma!
- Literary types will note the cute pun on sinful/cinnful!

9 – KIWI HEALTH CURE

Serving:

- Makes 2 glasses

Ingredients:

- Half a honeydew melon
- 2 Large bunches of green grapes
- 2 juicy apples
- 2 peaches
- 2 kiwi fruits

Instructions:

- Remove melon from skin and peel kiwi fruits
- Leave the skins on the rest, (but do remove the pips from apples and stones from peaches)
- Juice all of the ingredients
- Serve immediately over ice

Talking Points:

- What a nice, cool, refreshing drink, with a taste that seems to combine strawberry, pineapple, and nectarine – and how incredibly healthy
- The kiwifruit is full of flavour and will add a kick to your drink
- Avoid kiwi fruits that are too hard. Store unripe kiwis at room temperature until skin indents slightly when touched
- Kiwifruit has more vitamin C than the same amount of oranges, as much potassium as bananas, and four times as much fibre as celery
- This zestful drink also contains peaches, good for irritated stomachs, reduce high blood pressure and protect against cancer and heart disease
- Grapes fight carcinogens, lower blood pressure and relieve the symptoms of arthritis. Apples are an ideal antioxidant, good for cleansing and the digestive system
- This recipe is a good immune-system booster and is ideal for a hangover
- In fact, it's no bad thing to experiment with adding kiwifruit to all fruit smoothies or any refreshing drink to get a real boost that's tasty and healthy

10 – SUNDOWNER

I drank a delicious alcohol-free 'Sundowner' in Rick's Café, Negril, Jamaica, sometimes said to be the most dangerous bar in the world because it's perched atop a cliff which unwary customers have been known to dive off. Having been tipped off about the dangers I decided to keep a clear head!

Serving:

- Serves one

Ingredients:

- 30 mls white grape juice
- 30 mls pineapple juice
- 40 mls cold sparkling water
- Fresh mint sprig for garnishing

Instructions:

- Pour the ingredients into a wine glass with ice
- Stir and garnish it with the mint sprigs
- Serve chilled

Talking Points:

- A sundowner is normally understood to be an alcoholic drink taken after completing the day's work, usually at sundown
- Typically a modern sundowner contains Malibu Rum, Pineapple Juice and a couple of dashes of Angostura Bitters
- This non-alcoholic variant may not be as potent but it's not a bad substitute if you're on your way home from work and have a drive ahead of you

11 – JOYRIDE JIGGER

I first drank this in Barbados, at Sharkey's beach bar, and loved it so much I got the basic recipe from the barman who gave it me with some reluctance. I try to avoid taking alcohol while I'm soaking up the sun and this sensational drink is good enough reason to quit the demon booze forever!

Serving:

- Serves five generously

Ingredients:

- 250 mls cream of coconuts
- 500 mls chilled pineapple juice
- 350 mls chilled ginger ale

Instructions:

- In small punch bowl, stir together the cream of coconut and pineapple juice until well mixed
- Stir ginger ale in gently and serve immediately

Talking points:

- I was surprised how simple the recipe was for such a full, fizzy, fruity totally tropical taste
- Mind you anything cool tastes nice on a Barbados beach!
- And what, by the way, is a jigger? Technically, it's a small measure of liquor – but this Joyride is probably

so-called because it's so good, it makes you want to get up and dance a jig!

12 - ASTORIA DELUXE

One consumed at the wonderful Astoria, Lucerne, Switzerland, and the taste is never forgotten, although the original name is, so I've named it after the hotel. I reckon it must have been made something like this.

Serving:

- One generous serving

Ingredients:

- 90 mls orange juice
- 60 mls pineapple juice
- 350 mls kiwi syrup
- 4 strawberries

- 2 tbsp melons

Instructions:

- Blend until smooth
- Add half a glassful of crushed ice, and blend again briefly

Talking point

- For the want of a better name, let's call this after this ultra-modern hotel of fond memory
- It is a variant on the familiar combination of orange and pineapple but it is both delicious and different – and very health-giving

13 - GREEN KIWI WINE

Serving:

- Enough to fill a wine bottle

Ingredients:

- 500 mls grape juice
- 4 kiwi fruits, peeled and sliced
- 1 cup watermelon, peeled, seeded and cubed
- 1 lime, thinly sliced
- 45 mls non-alcoholic cider
- ¼ cup sugar

Instructions:

- Combine all ingredients in large jug, stirring to crush some of the fruit
- Cover and refrigerate overnight to let the flavours blend naturally
- Serve with added kiwi fruit

Talking Points:

- This may not be wine in the official sense but you'll find it's got a zesty kick and a subtle flavour!
- Delicious on a hot day and full of antioxidants

14 – BANANA AND HONEY SMOOTHIE

Serving:

- Two glasses

Ingredients:

- 150 mls of milk
- 2 large bananas
- 150 mls plain yoghurt
- 15 mls honey
- A pinch of cinnamon

Instructions:

- Throw everything in a blender and mix until smooth, velvety and frothy

Talking Points:

- Here is a basic smoothie that even a child could make and certainly every child will adore it. It is a great way to start the day
- It is ideal for using up old bananas and, in fact, different fruit can be added to give variations of taste, which is a good idea if you're going to start every day off like this

15 - CINDERELLA COCKTAIL

I was served a fantastic zero-proof Cinderella at St George's Hotel, near Pafos, Cyprus, when enjoying a package holiday there. They served a different non-alcoholic cocktail everyday and one like this was the drink I liked best.

Serving:

- Makes one cocktail

Ingredients:

- 30 mls lemon juice
- 30 mls orange juice
- 30 mls pineapple juice
- 60 mls ginger ale
- Dash of grenadine

- Pineapple and orange slices for garnish

Instructions

- Pour the juices into a cocktail shaker with ice cubes. Shake well
- Strain into a chilled collins glass filled with ice
- Garnish with the slices of pineapple or orange

Talking Points:

- The taste of tropical fruit comes to life in this refreshing mocktail, the non-alcoholic equivalent of the famous Cinderella Cocktail
- If you'd like a more elegant looking Cinderella, cut all of the juices and ginger ale in half and serve it in a chilled cocktail glass

16 – PASSATA APPERITIF

Serving:

Serves 4

Ingredients:

- 300mls passata sauce
- Juice of 2 limes – or lime juice from bottle
- ¼ nutmeg, grated
- 3 pinches of sugar
- 1 pinch of salt
- 1 pinch of chilli powder

Instructions:

- Place the passata, lime juice, nutmeg, salt and chilli powder in a large bowl and stir well
- Place in the fridge. Get a cold glass and slightly wet the rim
- Dip into the sugar
- Pour the mixture into the glass and decorate with a cherry and slice of orange
- Serve chilled

Talking Points:

- Passata is made from ripe tomatoes that have been puréed and sieved to remove the skin and seed.
- Make this colourful Italian-style cocktail to serve before a dinner party – the lime, chilli and tomato really give you a buzz
- And you do find your appetite has been stimulated!

17 - NETTLE BEER

I first experienced this way back at a drive-in about halfway between Clinton Ridge and Oak Ridge, on Highway 61, overlooking the Clinch River, where it was being sold in bottles, having been made locally from nettles collected on the banks of the river. Sadly I've never seen it on sale since that time, so decided to make it myself and discovered this old English recipe thanks to the British Lending Library.

Serving:

- Makes lots

Ingredients:

- 900 g young nettle tops
- 3.8 ltrs of water
- 230 g of brown or demarrara sugar
- 7.5 g of fresh yeast
- Small piece of toast
- 7.5 g of ground ginger

Instructions:

- Boil the nettle tops in the water for half an hour in a very large pan or   cauldron
- Strain and add sugar, stirring to dissolve
- Stir in the ginger and pour mixture into a sterile container
- Spread the yeast onto the toast and float on the surface of the nettle liquid
- Cover and leave for about 3 days at a constant room temperature
- Strain again and put into clean, strong screw top beer

Talking Points:

- This is an easy recipe to follow and creates a delightfully unusual beer, which can be drunk after a couple of days before it has become mildly alcoholic. It is very cheap to make and follows a traditionally English recipe
- Before hops were widely used in the 17th century many plants were used to flavour the ale including nettles. It was also thought to help alleviate rheumatic pain, gout and asthma
- Nettle has a long history as a herbal remedy. It is rich in chlorophyll and is a good source of beta carotene, tannins, iron, calcium, potassium and many other minerals. It is also rich in vitamin A, C and E
- Some people do find it a strong diuretic – something to make them pass water. Beware!

18 – RIO HOT CHOCOLATE

The best I've ever tasted was at the famous Bar Do Gomez, Rio De Janiero, an old Brazilian boteco, which hadn't changed since the Twenties and was just about the very incarnation of what every South American bar should look like. I thought it the most romantic cafe in Rio, if not in the world, and have never forgotten the rich taste and aroma of the hot chocolate consumed there one early morning, surrounded by serious locals drinking black coffee, smoking fat cigars and intently reading their Correio Braziliense.

Serving:

- Makes four cups

Ingredients:

- 1 ½ cups coffee
- 1 cup half-and-half cream
- 1 cup boiling water
- ¼ cup sugar
- 30 g chocolate
- 5 mls vanilla extract
- ½ tsp cinnamon
- Dash salt

Instructions:

- In a large pan melt the solid chocolate, the sugar and the salt.
- Stir in boiling water and continue to heat until the mixture is well blended and hot
- Add the coffee, the cream and stir well
- Finish by adding the vanilla and the cinnamon and pour into mugs
- Add a dollop of whipped cream

Talking Points:

- A drink popular in Brazil with a beautiful rich velvety taste
- And the best I've ever tasted was at the famous Bar Do Gomez, Rio De Janiero
- All the family will love this. Try it for a heavenly mid-morning pick-me up

19 - BANANA SLUSH

Serving:

Serves about 50

Ingredients:

- 500 mls lemonade
- 400 mls orange juice
- 4 cups sugar
- 6 cups water
- 5 bananas
- 1 ltr pineapple juice
- 500 mls ginger ale

Instructions:

- Boil the sugar with the cups of water in a large saucepan for 3 minutes. Allow to cool

- Mash the bananas in a blender and combine with the orange juice, lemonade, pineapple juice, and bananas in a large bowl. Add sugar syrup; blend well
- Freeze the mixture for at least 24 hours
- Remove from freezer 1 hour before serving
- Using a fork, break frozen punch into smaller pieces
- Add ginger ale
- Continue blending until slushy
- Serve in tall glasses with added lemons

Talking Points:

- This is ideal for a big children's party because if makes a lot, very easily and without much in the way of equipment
- All ages will enjoy this, however

20 - MOUNTAIN MALOTIRA

I first drank Greek Mountain tea, this deliciously warming and pungent brew, on Crete where the common name for it is 'Malotira". The best cup I actually ever had was in a small café overlooking the square, in the charming, inland village of Peza, best known for its wine but clearly very near a rich source of sideris!

Ingredients and preparation:

It's made pretty much in the same way as ordinary tea, using the dried leaves and flowers of Sideritis plants otherwise known as ironwort.

Talking Points:

- Aptly named Mountain Tea because the plant used to make it is found on rocky slopes at great height and only in Greece is it cultivated
- Every region of Greece has its own name for the brew, such as "Olympos tea," and "Parnassos tea," depending on the name of the mountain where it grows.
- Outside Greece, it is sold as "Greek Mountain Tea," or "Greek Mountain Shepherd's Tea," this last because Greek shepherds, tending their flocks, would use the plants to make a brew
- Enormously popular in Greece, it's used most often in winter to ward off colds, aches, and pains
- It is used for colds, respiratory problems, digestion, the immune system, mild anxiety, and as an anti-oxidant. It is also used as an anti-inflammatory and to reduce fever

21- GOGI BERRY BADOIT

I drank this one shimmering afternoon whilst sitting on the pavement terrace of the well-named La Belle Epoque, in Aix-en-Provence, listening to a quartet playing jazz of the Django Reinhardt variety. The drink seemed just right for the occasion.

Serving:

Several glasses

Ingredients:

- 1 bottle Badoit
- 1 bottle gogi berries

Instructions:

Blend the two liquids to taste, approximately in equal measures.

Talking Points:

- This beautiful and little known drink, outside of France, is simplicity itself
- Badoit and Gogi berries seem to go very well together, as I discovered when being served it in Aix-en-Provenance
- Badoit is a brand of lightly sparkling mineral water obtained from natural sources at Saint-Galmier, France, from a depth of more than 100 metres in granite. The

water is naturally carbonated on its journey through the subterranean gas deposits
- Many years ago local physicians were already prescribing Badoit for its curative powers, and the remains of Roman baths can still be seen at the spring
- Its hint of sodium bicarbonate is said to aid the digestive system
- Nutritionists and dieticians are enthusiastic about the antioxidant qualities of gogi berries, or wolfberries as they are sometimes called, and they have been termed a superfruit

22 – WIENER KRACHERL

I drank this, before going on the piste, in the beautiful 17th-century Hotel Lebzelter, Zell Am See, Austria, strongly recommended as a refreshing drink by one of the lederhosen-clad barmen. Later, après ski, he recommended something much stronger.

Serving:

Several generous glasses

Ingredients:

- 1 bottle Raspberry Kracherl, mixed with a load of ice

Instructions:

- Pour into a glass over ice
- Insert slices of lemon for a certain added piquancy

Talking Points:

- The typical Wiener Kracherl is an Austrian classic and one you should not miss out on if you go to this country. Unfortunately, it is difficult to obtain it anywhere else
- In 1912 in a far corner of Austria, the Windisch family started to make soft drinks with their brand name, Kracherl. The name comes from the crashing noise, which generates the carbonic acid while opening the bottle
- In addition to the pure taste of the raspberry Kracherl, there are other delicious flavours, for example orange, or Ribisel, a blending of fruit punch. They are available carbonated or non-carbonated.
- For those who want alcohol, it is popular to blend Ribisel with white or red wine in a half-litre glass - or to mix un-carbonated kracherls with beers

23 – PINK CHAMPAGNE

Serving:

Serves up to 6 cocktail glasses

Ingredients:

- 200 mls grape juice
- 200 mls water
- 300 mls orange juice
- Bottle ginger ale
- Grenadine syrup

Instructions:

- Mix first 4 ingredients
- Chill in a fridge for half an hour
- Divide the mixture between 4 champagne glasses
- Top up each with ginger ale and stir gently
- Add grenadine syrup to taste and stir again

Talking Points:

- This delicious 'champagne' is very easy to make and tastes remarkably refreshing
- It is sparkling like the real thing, which, as everyone knows, has to be produced from grapes that grow in the Champagne appellation of France, although increasingly these days it is being used as a generic term for sparkling wine

24 – GUAVA PALAVER

I encountered this potent little number in the elegant surroundings of The Lounge at Nobu, Honolulu, a bar very famous for its cocktails. Like all such places, it does a nice selection of zero-proof drinks if you ask.

Serving:

Makes one generous drink

Ingredients:

- 150 mls guava juice
- 350 mls rose water

Instructions:

- Pour the ingredients into a cocktail shaker filled with ice
- Shake well and strain into a chilled cocktail glass
- Garnish with a lemon or lime

Talking Points:

- No palaver at all making this delicious alcohol-free cocktail which is oozing health-giving qualities
- Guava has a taste all of its own, although some people think it tastes a bit like pear

- Guava juice is very popular in Hawaii, Cuba, Costa Rica, Puerto Rico, Colombia, Venezuela, Egypt, Mexico and South Africa
- Guava fruit is often prepared in fruit salads and is rich in fibre, vitamins A and C, folic acid, and potassium, copper and manganese
- A single fruit contains about four times the amount of vitamin C as an orange and is also a valuable source of vitamin A and B, nicotinic acid, phosphorous, potassium and iron
- Guavas are also low in fat and calories, with only about 25 calories per fruit and are said lower cholesterol, protect the heart and are good for the immune system

25 – LEMON & PAEROA

I had my first in the Fringe Bar, Wellington, a lively place well known for it comedy acts, in a rather bohemian district of Wellington. The locals did find it immensely funny that here was a drink quite unknown to me, a so-called drinks expert!

Serving:

You'll get plenty of drinks out of a bottle

Instructions:

Buy it by the bottle when Down Under.

Talking Points:

- Lemon & Paeroa, according to its own witty advertising slogan, is World famous in New Zealand
- New Zealanders all over the world know all about L&P, although most of the rest of the world has yet to hear about it
- It was made from a natural spring in the North Island town of Paeroa, which is situated about an hour south east of Auckland
- It tastes delicious and something like a lemon squash mixed with a kind of root beer.
- You'll probably have to go to the sub-continent to see it being sold, although it can be ordered on line.

26 – GRANNIE ANNIE'S ORANGE SQUASH

This was made for me many years ago by a girlfriend's mother, Annie, who spent most of her life in Easton, Fairfield County, Connecticut, a little place better known for its apple drinks than for its orange squash.

Serving:

Serves 2

Ingredients:

- 3 oranges minced or blended
- 60 g citric acid
- 2 k sugar
- 2.5 ltrs boiling water

Instructions:

- Bring oranges and water to boil
- Turn off heat and add citric acid and sugar stir until sugar is dissolved
- Leave to cool, then strain and bottle
- Dilute with cold water to taste

Talking Points:

- This is a recipe Annie taught me many years ago.
- It's simple to do and the taste is simple too.
- A lovely orange squash without any additional under-taste and very nice for the whole family on a hot day – and remarkably health giving

27 - CHAI TEA

The best cup that's ever passed my lips was served at the Cha Bar, which was described to me as Delhi's most prestigious tea lounge - at Connaught Place's Statesman Tower. Part of the Oxford Bookstore, it was amazing how well tea and good literature seemed to complement each other.

Serving:

Makes a large teapot full

Ingredients:

- 4 tsp black tea
- 1 cinnamon stick
- 5 g fennel seeds
- 6 cardamom pods, bruised
- 150 mls of milk
- 750 mls of water
- Sugar to taste

Instructions:

- Break the cinnamon stick in half and add to the saucepan with fennel seeds and cardamom pods
- Add water to the saucepan and bring to the boil over high heat.
- Add tea and keep boiling for 1 minute.
- Add milk and bring to the boil again. Add sugar to taste and stir well.
- Strain tea into a teapot and then strain again

Talking Points:

- You've never tasted tea until you've tasted Chai - which is becoming increasingly popular in cafes around the world
- Originating from the Indian subcontinent, it is made from brewing black tea leaves with a mixture of aromatic spices, these being in this recipe, cardamom, cinnamon and fennel seeds, but in others can include cloves, pepper and ginger
- The amount of sugar you add is optional but remember the sweetness is needed to bring out the full flavours of the spices
- The word Chai is actually the name for tea in many countries
- Offering tea rather than alcoholic drinks to visitors is the cultural norm in India. Tea has also entered the common idiom so much so that the term "Chai-Panii" (Tea and Water) usually refers to wages, tips or even bribery!

28 - WASSAIL PUNCH

Serving:

Serves 6-8

Ingredients:

- 1.2 ltrs apple juice
- 250mls orange juice
- 3-4 cinnamon sticks
- 4 cloves
- Zest from ½ lemon
- 4 apples
- 1 ½ cups brown sugar
- 1 cup red grape juice
- ½ teaspoon ground cinnamon
- ¼ teaspoon ground all spice
- ¼ teaspoon ground cardamom
- ½ teaspoon ground ginger

Instructions:

- Preheat your oven to 175 degrees C
- In a large sauce pan, pour in 2 pints of apple juice
- Add the cinnamon sticks, lemon zest and cloves and bring to a simmer over low heat
- Take the apples and score with a knife before placing in a baking dish. Cover with one cup of brown sugar, 1/4 cup of orange juice, and all of the red grape juice. Cover baking dish and place in oven, cooking for 30 minutes
- While apples are baking, place remaining sugar and spices into the sauce pan, ensuring it's well mixed
- When apples are baked, place entire contents of baking dish into sauce pan and allow to cook over a low heat for another 30-40 minutes

Talking Points:

- This non-alcoholic version of a traditional English drink is a sumptuous and aromatic brew of apple and orange juice infused with hand-blended spices
- Serve hot as a simple and easy option for festive occasions or when relaxing by a log file for a deep, rich and spicy taste
- For the record, wassail is an ancient greeting used at holiday times, coming from the Anglo-Saxon phrase *waes hael*, often used as a toast - meaning, be hale or good health

29 - BANANA AND PEANUT BUTTER SMOOTHIE

Serving:

Serves two

Ingredients:
- 1 Banana
- 300 mls semi-skimmed milk
- 15 mls smooth peanut butter
- 5 mls honey
- Garnish with a pinch of cinnamon
- Decorate with a strawberry

Instructions:

- Peel and slice banana and freeze for a couple of hours
- Blend banana slices, milk, peanut butter and honey until smooth
- Pour mixture into glasses
- Garnish and decorate

Talking Points:

- What could be more nutritional than this delicious blending of banana and peanut butter!
- Peanut butter contains folate (converting to folic acid in the body), vitamin E, magnesium and resveratrol (the anti-ageing antioxidant), all nutrients associated with reduced risk of heart disease
- Magnesium is also associated with reduced risk of diabetes
- Peanut butter also contains a small amount of zinc, a mineral important for healing and strengthening the immune system

30 – MALTA

I came across it at its delicious best whilst staying at a gem of a place, sitting on the terrace, watching the sun go down over Marigot Bay - The Inn On The Bay, St Lucia, where all dreams seem possible

Serving:

Can be bought in bottles in many countries

Ingredients:

Barley, hops, water, soda

Talking Points:

- Malta (also called young beer, children's beer, or wheat soda) originated in Germany as Malzbier ("malt beer")
- These days, it's a non-alcoholic, carbonated malt beverage, brewed from barley, hops, and water much like beer but without the fermentation and a delicious alternative to the usual varieties of soda, pop and colas sometimes branded as Champagne Cola
- It has similar dark brown colour to stout but is very sweet, tasting rather like molasses
- Latin Americans often drink malta mixed with condensed or evaporated milk
- Nowadays, a great deal of malta is brewed in the Caribbean and can be purchased in areas with substantial Caribbean populations but is also popular in many parts of Africa like Nigeria, Chad, Ghana, Cameroon, and in the Indian Ocean
- Malta is high in B vitamins

31 - MANGO LASSI

I always used to drink Mango Lassi at my favourite London curry house - the newly fashionable Aladin Brick Lane, a place apparently now favoured by Prince Charles when he fancies something gently spicy. I have to say I've never seen him there, though! Certainly Lassi has a cooling, soothing effect to offset the heat of the strongest of curries – the hottest known to me, by the way, being Satan's Ashes. Leave it alone!

Serving:

Serves two

Ingredients:

- ¼ cup plain low-fat yogurt
- ½ teaspoon freshly-squeezed lemon juice
- ½ cup fresh mango pulp
- ½ cup cold water
- 30-60 mls honey or sugar
- Standard-size ice cubes

Preparation:

- Take the fresh mango, peel and remove the flesh from the pith
- Cut into small pieces
- Do not waste any of the juices
- Blend the yogurt, lemon juice, mango pulp, water, and honey or sugar for 2 to 3 minutes or until a mixture starts to form
- Add the ice and blend until frothy
- Alternatively, you could buy the mango juice ready prepared

Talking Points:

- Mango Lassi is a traditional South Asian non-alcoholic beverage - and one of the most popular in Northern India and in Indian restaurants around the world
- It's something like a cross between a smoothie and a milk shake and is creamy and delicious!
- When choosing a mango, pick one that is plump and fragrant. Canned or frozen mango may be substituted

32 - PRICKLY PEAR BONANZA

Serving:

Serves 2

Ingredients:

- ½ cup crushed ice
- 30 mls freshly-squeezed lime juice
- 30 mls undiluted frozen limeade
- 60 mls pear juice
- I large dash grenadine
- 30 mls prickly pear cactus juice
- 15 g granulated sugar or corn syrup

- Lime wedges for garnish

Instructions:

- Blend crushed ice, lime juice, pear juice, grenadine, prickly pear juice, and sugar or corn syrup
- Cover and mix
- Add sugar to taste

Talking Points:

- Prickly Pear Bonanaza is a zero-proof version of the increasingly popular Prickly Pear Marguerita, generally made with Tequila and Cointreau
- Prickly Pear, one of the latest super foods, takes its name from its pear-like shape and size
- This fruit comes from any of several varieties of cacti and is also called cactus pear
- It has a melon-like aroma and a sweet but rather bland flavour

33 – STRAWBERRY SURPRISE

I had one such in Paris, in the beautifully baroque ambience of La Delaville Café, and paid a fortune for it, as you do on or around the Champs Elysees – but fortunately I was on expenses!

Serving:

Makes one delicious drink

Ingredients:

- 30 mls fresh lime juice
- 90 mls fresh strawberries
- 5 g sugar
- Cracked ice

Instructions:

- Fill lime juice, strawberries, and sugar into a blender
- Blend until smooth, then add the cracked ice and blend again until smooth
- Pour into a chilled cocktail glass
- Garnish with whole strawberry

Talking Points:

- This is the perfect drink for everyone who just loves the taste of Strawberry Daiquiri, but prefers not to drink alcohol
- The fresh and juicy non- alcoholic strawberry daiquiri is a wonderful cocktail for a hot summer day
- Because of the heady strawberry flavour you won't even notice the missing alcohol

34 – BIRTHDAY CELEBRATION

Serving:

Makes one birthday treat!

Ingredients:

- 45 mls lime juice
- 30 mls sugar syrup
- 15 mls raspberry syrup
- 10 mls grenadine syrup
- 90 mls soda water

Instructions:

- Rim a wine glass with lime/caster sugar, add a spiral of lime, and fill with crushed ice
- Stir lime juice and syrups together and strain into the glass
- Add the soda and sprinkle the grenadine on
- Garnish with strawberries

Talking Points:

- What better zero-proof drink could you wish for on that special day you toast yourself

- And all your friends will love it

35 – PEACH PUNCH

Serving:

Makes plenty for everyone

Ingredients:

- 1.4 ltr peach nectar
- 600 mls orange juice
- ½ cup brown sugar
- 3 3-inch cinnamon sticks
- ½ tsp cloves
- 30 mls lime juice

Instructions:

- Combine peach nectar, orange juice and brown sugar in a large saucepan
- Tie cinnamon and cloves in a small cheesecloth bag. Drop into saucepan
- Heat slowly, stirring constantly, until sugar dissolves. Simmer for 10 minutes
- Stir in lime juice
- Serve in hot mugs garnished with lemon and summer fruit

Talking Points:

- Non-alcoholic punch is very popular in German-speaking countries and this one is guaranteed to warm the cockles of your heart!
- It's good to drink this one on festival occasions, whether it's Christmas morning or on the eve of Eid - but it is good to warm you on all those cold winter days

I was served something very like this in Milan, at the Caffe Cova, right next to La Scala, founded in 1817 and one of Ernest Hemingway's favourites. I'd gone in to partake of the fabled coffee but saw someone drinking this colourful concoction and knew I had to try it before I did anything else.

Serving:

Makes two generous drinks

Ingredients:

- 60 mls mango juice
- 30 mls pineapple juice
- 30 mls orange juice
- 15 mls strawberry syrup
- 60 mls dry ginger ale

Instructions:

- Shake the juice and syrup, and strain into an ice-filled wine goblet
- Add the ginger ale
- Garnish with seasonal fruit, and sprinkle with grated nutmeg.
- Serve with straws

Talking Point:

- A jazzy drink popular with all ages, and capable of infinite of variations

38 – SIGUIENTE

I drank a variant of this at Eurostar's Grand Marina in Barcelona's Ciutat Vella neighbourhood, where I spent all day looking out over the harbour contemplating which delicious drink to have next.

Serving:

As much as you like, just double up on all the ingredients

Ingredients:

- 2 parts orange juice
- 3 parts lemon lime Soda
- 1 parts Lime Juice
- Lemon slices
- Mint leaves

Instructions:

- Fill a shaker with ice cubes and add all ingredients

- Shake and strain into a chilled highball glass filled with ice cubes
- Garnish with lemon and mint

Talking Points:

- 'Siguente' is Spanish for the next one and a cocktail of this order is very commonly found in cafés on Barcelona's Rambla
- It certainly is a refreshing drink for a day in a hot Spanish city

39 - SCRAPPLE FROM THE APPLE

'Scrapple from the Apple' is a Be-bop composition by Charlie Parker, written in 1947, and this drink, a wonderful version of which I was privileged to consume in Desmond's Tavern, on Park Avenue South, New York, is apparently named after the great Jazz tenor saxophonist

Serving:

Serves four

Ingredients:

- 250 mls apples – peeled and sliced
- 120 mls pineapple - slices
- 250 mls orange juice
- 90 mls lemon juice
- Sugar to taste

Instructions:

- Mix the fruit juices with the sugar until it is dissolved.
- Add the slices of apple and pineapple and chill.
- Serve in Collins glasses and garnish with a slice of orange

Talking Point:

- And by the way if you're ever in Desmond's treat yourself to one of his delicious Coby Jack hamburgers, if you're feeling hungry!

40 –ALGIERS STRUT

I'd taken the ferry across the Mississippi one hot, swampy afternoon, and came to the famous Old Point Bar in Algiers, which advertised itself as 'the most filmed bar in the South'. I didn't think much of what the local young people were drinking, until I tried it – and then wow!

Serving:

2 long drinks

Ingredients:

- Half bottle Coca-Cola
- Half bottle orange juice

Instructions:

- Fill ¼ of tall glass with ice
- Pour over the orange juice, then the Coke
- Stir gently to mix

Talking Points:

- This is a drink that comes from the Algiers of New Orleans, not the African country
- It's a stimulating drink for hot, sunny, swampy days. It's refreshingly different and quite a daring combination, really

42 – HORCHATA

Serving:

Serves 2

Ingredients:

- 1 cup uncooked white long-grain rice
- 5 cups water
- 75 mls milk
- 7.5 mls vanilla extract
- ½ tablespoon ground cinnamon
- ¾ cup white sugar
- Cinnamon powder sprinkles or chocolate powder

Instructions:

- Pour the rice and water into the bowl of a blender; blend until the rice just begins to break up, about 1 minute
- Let rice and water stand at room temperature for a minimum of 3 hours
- Strain the rice water into a pitcher and discard the rice
- Stir the milk, vanilla, cinnamon, and sugar into the rice water
- Chill and stir before serving over ice 2/3 cup white sugar
- Top with cinnamon powder sprinkles or chocolate powder (or both)

Talking Points:

- This delicious Mexican cinnamon rice milk is a delicate and subtle taste
- Use rice milk, which is lighter than ordinary milk, if you like the flavour of it
- There are versions of horchata that use plain milk (whole or skim), coconut milk or condensed milk

42 – THAT'S A PLENTY

Serving:

Serves 1

Ingredients:

- 1 small cucumber
- 2 tomatoes
- 1 stick celery
- 1 orange
- Worcester sauce

Instructions:

- Collect the juices from the cucumber, tomato, celery and orange using a juice extractor
- Season with Worcester sauce to taste

Talking Points:

- Here's a drink to take mid-morning instead of a snack
- It's easy and quick and a real pick-me-up with far fewer calories than coffee and biscuits
- It's delicious when seasoned to taste with salt, pepper and Worcestershire sauce
- Good for a hangover or part of a detox diet

43– WHITE HORSE WONDER

I consumed a very special hangover cure, one Sunday morning in the early-1980s, in the famous White Horse Inn in Manhattan's West Village - where the great Welsh poet, Dylan Thomas, met his unfortunate end after downing 18 glasses of assorted alcohol. Norman Mailer, Anais Nin and an A-Z of other writers, from the proprietors of new journalism to beatnik poets, spent time here as did I – lots of it.

Serving:

Makes one hangover cure

Ingredients:

- 60 ml olive oil
- 1 raw egg yolk
- Salt and pepper to taste
- 20 mls of tomato ketchup
- A dash of Tabasco and Worcestershire
- Lemon juice (or vinegar)

Instructions:

- Combine all the ingredients in a shaker and add the lemon juice last to avoid curdling
- Alternatively use a blender

Talking Points:

- I asked the barman for something for a hangover, figuring he would know, and this is what he came up with. Pity Dylan Thomas didn't drink it instead
- The egg yolk contains N-acetyl-cysteine (NAC), an amino acid that helps to drive out the toxins acquired from drink and tobacco. Tomato ketchup provides bioflavonoids which are an excellent source of antioxidants to help boost the immune system
- Consuming fruit or fruit juice while hungover can increase energy, replaces vitamins and nutrients and has been shown to speed up the body's process of getting rid of toxins. Fruits and fruit juices therefore can help decrease the intensity of hangover symptoms, so any of the fruit cocktails in this book would also help
- Bananas in particular help to replenish many essential salts. Also drink lots of water, at least twice the amount of water to alcohol and take some vitamin C and some sugar because alcohol lowers your blood sugar levels
- Avoid aspirin as the alcohol has probably already made your stomach lining rather sensitive and you don't want to make yourself sick

44 – HAWAII ROYAL

I discovered a delightful version of this very simple but never-to-be forgotten drink at the Royal Hawaiian Hotel in Waikiki, where it was a perfect way to stay cool while looking out over the shimmering bay over to Diamond Head and watch the sun go down.

Serving:

Serves one long drink

Ingredients:

- 1 banana
- 500 mls pineapple juice
- 90 mls coconut milk
- 15 g sugar

Instructions:

- Slice the banana, and place it in a blender with the pineapple juice, coconut milk and a tablespoon of white sugar
- Blend the ingredients together until the consistency is smooth, and then pour it into a large glass

Talking Points:

- Here's a great mixed drink that combines some fresh fruit with a tropical-tinged beverage
- Whoever thought of combining banana, coconut and pineapple was a genius

45 – MINT MANHATTAN

I am not sure what the original name for this was but I came across it in Manhattan so will give it that name, although aware, of course, a Manhattan is commonly a cocktail made with whiskey, sweet vermouth, and bitters. I was in the Plunge at Hotel Gansevoort where the rooftop views over the city were mesmerising and the drinks intoxicating even zero-proof.

Serving:

Serves 1

Ingredients:

- 20 mls peppermint syrup
- 2 - 3 mint leaves
- 150 mls tonic water

Instructions:

- Place the mint leaves into a large highball glass, and pour in peppermint syrup
- Press with a bar spoon

- Add a scoop of crushed ice, fill with tonic water, and stir.

Talking Points:

- This is a very nice drink, very simple to make and one that really peps up your palate.
- Mint is as good for you as it is pleasant to ingest and is widely used as a healthy form of flavouring I food and drinks
- There are many types of mint including, apple mint, water mint, horsemint, pineapple mint, orange mint, pennyroyal and spearmint and, of course peppermint, used in toothpaste, chewing gum, mouthwash, soaps and medicines
- The barman prescribed as a cure for indigestion and it certainly worked for me

46 – BANANA MALT

Serves:

1 Smoothie

Ingredients:

- 2 bananas (ripe, cut into chunks roughly mashed)
- 2 tbsps chocolate syrup
- 2 tbsps milk
- 420 mls vanilla ice cream

- 1 tbsp malted milk powder

Instructions:

- Place mashed banana, syrup, milk, ice cream& malted milk powder in blender
- Blend on medium-high speed until all ingredients are thoroughly blended and smooth

Talking Points:

- This is a very healthy drink based on the well-known product Horlicks, whose sleep-inducing qualities are well known
- London pharmacist James Horlick brought his ideas for a wheat and malt-based nutritional dried milk drink to America where he patented it in 1887
- Despite its origins as a health food for infants and invalids, travellers and explorers   appreciated its portable and non-perishable qualities, and the popularity of malted milk spread widely

47 – BRIGHT LAMP SMOOTHIE

Serving:

Serves two

Ingredients:

- 4 rings of fresh pineapple
- 1 mango
- 5 apples
- 1 lime
- Slice of ginger (to taste)
- 4 good scoops of fresh yoghurt

Instructions:

- Prepare and freeze the mango and pineapple.
- Add to a blender followed by the juiced apples, lime and ginger.
- Add the yoghurt, blend well and serve immediately.

Talking Points:

- This drink is named after the initial letters of its ingredients: lime, apple, mango, pineapple – and it is a shining example of a smoothie
- The combination of pineapple, mango, lime, ginger and yoghurt is   rather special

48 – SALSA DRINK

Serving:

Serves 6

Ingredients:

- Carton of tomato juice
- ½ a Red Pepper
- ½ a Stick of Celery
- ¼ of a Red Onion
- ½ a Clove of Garlic
- Fresh Green or Red Chilli (to taste)
- Juice of 1 Lime
- Small Bunch of Fresh Coriander

Instructions:

- Wash and prepare all the ingredients then place them in a blender and whisk to a rich consistency
- Garnish with a lime

Talking Points:

- A salsa is a sauce, and the word usually refers to the spicy, often tomato-based, hot sauces typical of Spanish or Mexican cuisine
- This little number is a drink with the taste and ingredients of a salsa. You won't be drinking this in large measures but savouring it before or with a Mediterranean meal

49- GINGER TEA

Serving:

Makes 2 cups

Ingredients:

- 300 mls water
- 1 inch fresh ginger root grated or slice

- 2 cloves
- 4 cardamoms
- Pinch of fennel seeds
- A small piece of cinnamon stick
- 2 teaspoons of tea leaves or 1 tea bag

Instruction:

- Crush all spices using pestle and mortar to bring out the flavour of the spices
- Place water, ginger and all spices in a pot and bring to boil
- Cover and lower the heat to allow it to simmer for about 10 minutes
- Add tea leaves and bring it to a gentle boil, then allow it to simmer for about 10 minutes
- Add milk and bring to a gentle boil
- Remove from heat and add sugar or honey as desired
- Strain before serving!

Talking Points:

- You can vary the taste of this excellent drink by using different types of tea
- Experiment and discover which suits your taste buds best
- The Health Benefits of Tea are numerous
- According to the UK Tea Council, 4 cups of tea a day, taken with milk, provides significant amounts of the following nutrients:
- Approximately 17% of the recommended intake for calcium
- 5% for zinc
- 22% for Vitamin B2
- 5% for folic acid
- 5% for Vitamins B1 and B6

50 – ORANGE SHERBERT GINGER ALE

Serving:

Makes one serving

Ingredients:

- 250 mls ginger ale (regular or diet)
- 1 scoop orange sherbet - any flavour can be substituted

Instructions:

- Pour ginger ale in a glass and add a scoop of sherbet.
- Allow the sherbet to melt slightly then stir until mixed
- Garnish with slice of orange

Talking Points:

- This fun recipe is commonly used as a punch at parties
- For an alcoholic version: add a shot of gin to the mix for a refreshing and unique drink. The juniper and orange flavour of gin mixes perfectly with this concoction.

51 - LEMON SELZER

Believe it or not, I actually drank a version of this in the elegant surroundings of the lobby lounge of the Kowloon Shangri-La, Hong Kong, while waiting for a taxi to take me to the airport. I was feeling a bit off it ahead of my long flight and the barman was kind enough to make me this very pleasant-tasting stomach-settler

Serving:

Makes one drink

Ingredients:

- 3 thin slices of orange (peel on)
- 10 mls almond syrup

- 60 mls lemon lime soda
- 30 mls pink grapefruit juice
- 15 mls lemonade
- 20 mls seltzer water or club soda
- 2 dashes bitters

Instructions:

- Using a tablespoon, lightly crush the orange slices in a tall glass.
- Do not mash the oranges but crush them enough to release their flavour
- Add ¼ cup ice to the cup, fill with the remaining ingredients, and then stir lightly, keeping the orange slices at the bottom of the glass

Talking Points:

- Lemon lime soda gives a nice neutral taste and the addition of almond syrup to the oranges has an almost candy-like quality.
- Club soda and seltzer water, by the way, are essentially interchangeable.
- Strictly, seltzer is just water and carbon dioxide (made by pressurizing water with CO_2) and club soda may have some other minerals added (like salt).

52 – AFTERGLOW

I caressed this for a long time, and ultimately drank it, in the hallowed surroundings of the Long Bar of the Raffles Hotel – where else! – in Singapore. All the rest of my party were tossing back, like there was no tomorrow, the fabled Singapore Slings, which were practically invented here. But I still needed a clear head to put the finishing touches to a presentation I was giving next day, so I opted for this little number, which I reckon must have been made very much like the recipe below.

Serving:

Serves two

Ingredients:

- 4 cl Grenadine
- 12 cl of Pineapple juice
- 12 cl of Orange juice

Instructions:

- Mix all the ingredients in a cocktail shaker
- Pour the mixture into a highball glass containing some crushed ice
- Serve chilled, garnished with wedge of orange

Talking Points:

- The Afterglow is a cocktail that is tropical and sweet in nature
- It is a perfect beachside beverage and is equally at home on a hot summer day or evening

- It is also a relatively simple beverage to produce
- It's a perfect choice for the last delicious drink in this book. We hope you will have a wonderful afterglow – after every one of them!!

I do hope you have enjoyed this collection of some of my favourite drinks - and that it will bring you hours of pleasure!

Printed in Great Britain
by Amazon